CW00665412

OESTROGEN
THE KILLER IN OUR MIDST

Best wishes

Chris Woollams

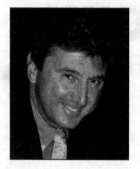

Chris has a degree in biochemistry and has formally studied both cancer and nutrition. Nowadays he is a tireless cancer researcher, with a magazine (**icon**) and several books to help people touched by cancer. He is much in demand as a speaker and has recently been in the USA and Australia apart from a tour with TV and media appearances all round Britain and Ireland.

OESTROGEN
THE KILLER IN OUR MIDST

How to combat the
biggest health threat today

CHRIS WOOLLAMS
M.A. (Oxon)

First published in March 2004 by:
Health Issues Ltd
The Elms, Radclive Road, Gawcott, Buckingham, MK18 4JB
Tel: 01280 815166
Fax: 01280 824655
E-mail: enquiries@iconmag.co.uk

Cover design by Jeremy Baker.

ISBN 0-9542968-3-4

Printed in England by Bath Press Ltd, Lower Bristol Road, Bath, BA2 3BL

For Julia and Renee, Peter and Richard,
Liz and Cathy
and all people who have hormonally
responsive cancers

IMPORTANT NOTICE

This info-book represents a review and an interpretation of a vast number of varied sources available to anyone on the subject of oestrogen and cancer.

Whilst the author has made every effort to ensure that the facts, information and conclusions are accurate and as up to date as possible at the time of publication, the author and publisher assume no responsibility.

The author is neither a fully qualified Health Practitioner nor a Doctor of Medicine and so is not qualified to give any advice on any medical matters. Cancer (and its related illnesses) is a very serious and very individual disease, and readers must consult with experts and specialists in the appropriate medical field before taking, or refraining from taking, any action.

This book and the advice contained are not intended as an alternative to such specialist advice, which should be sought for accurate diagnosis and before any course of treatment.

The author and the publisher cannot be held responsible for any action, or lack of action, that is taken by any reader as a result of information contained in the text of this book. Such action is taken entirely at the reader's own risk.

Nothing so needs reforming as other people's habits.

Mark Twain

CONTENTS

INTRODUCTION

Having researched the causes of cancer extensively for a number of years now, I want to make two points up front in this book:

1. I am convinced that in each of us, male or female, there is an 'oestrogen pool' and that whilst this may have normally declined in women with age, or been miniscule in men, nowadays it is abnormally high largely due in no small part to synthetic, man-made oestrogens and chemical toxins that mimic the action of oestrogen within our bodies.

2. This 'oestrogen pool' is causal to many rapidly growing cancers in both men and women. For example:

> prostate cancer
> colon cancer
> skin/melanoma cancer
> ovarian cancer
> endometrial cancer
> breast cancer
> and even some brain tumours.

Thirty or so years ago high levels of breast cancer in Israel were attributed to the pesticides DDT and Lindane. Unfortunately these chemicals were only banned for use in the West and not for worldwide sale, so you may, even today, consume them on your vegetables from third world countries where they are still used.

Dr Philippa Darbre of Reading University has shown

links between breast cancers and antiperspirants on a number of occasions. Swedish research recently showed that three quarters of perfumed products contained chemicals that once in the bloodstream formed DEHP, a toxic oestrogen mimic so dangerous it can cause the male offspring of pregnant women to have severe genital problems.

Pesticides, herbicides, antiperspirants and toiletries, perfumes and personal care products, household products like bleaches; fifty years ago the world produced just 1 million tonnes of chemicals; now that figure is 400 million tonnes, with little check on their safety.

The Royal Commission reported in 2002 that we commonly come into contact with 4000 ingredients, the majority of which are toxic and many are carcinogenic.

In November 2003 the WWF report studied the presence of 77 highly toxic chemicals in people in the UK. They found an average of 27 with the highest at 45. Pesticides like DDT and Lindane were there in our bloodstreams, as were highly dangerous PCBs and even PDBEs, used as flame-retardants in cars and furniture.

Yet we know for example, that **oestrogen has the ability to reduce oxygen levels in cells and set the scene for cancer to form.** For many years we have known **oestrogen also helps cancer cells to spread their message around the body.** Dr Ana Soto of Tufts

Cancer Research Center has also shown that chemicals, leaching in from her plastic research dishes, mimic the action of oestrogen and have the same effect.

HRT and the pill add enormous volumes of synthetic oestrogen to our women folk.

Our water and our food can raise the levels of our oestrogen pool too. Just recently the National Cancer Institute in the USA showed that obesity was linked to higher levels of oestrogen in the body and, although the study was done for women and breast cancer, you can bet it holds true for men and women and a host of cancers.

Meanwhile Cancer Research UK in 2003 told us that breast cancer was increasing by two per cent per year in Britain, while oestrogen levels in women were increasing faster. They argued that less babies, less breastfeeding, coupled with the use of synthetic oestrogen in the pill and HRT, caused much of the gain in the 'oestrogen pool' but that they were not sure of the full reasons. At **icon** we are. We wrote to them about oestrogen mimics and toxic chemicals.

By November 2003 Cancer Research UK was saying 'we do not know the cause of prostate cancer'. Yet there have been several studies showing clearly that localised oestrogen is implicated and it has long been known that oestrogen mimics cause genital problems, decreased sperm counts and are linked to prostate growth. In August 2003 in the Houston Cancer Center, Dr

Thomson published results that oestrogen turns the declining levels of testosterone in males into a highly dangerous substance called DHT. Again, chemicals that mimic the action of oestrogen are implicated.

Cancer Research UK also commented on Philippa Darbre's latest research. She showed that parabens, a preservative in antiperspirants, was found in breast cancer cells. Cancer Research stated that there was no research evidence that it was causal to cancer. Yet she has now produced several consistent studies.

Why is Europe's largest cancer charity in denial? Why does it, in effect, muddy the waters for people wishing to prevent cancer? Some would say it receives vast sums of money from pharmaceutical companies, many of which also have an interest in selling antiperspirants, toiletries and household products, the very substances that could be behind the upsurge in cancers in the Western world. Or maybe they genuinely don't know about all the research being conducted around the world showing the effects of chemicals on our health.

Several studies, the latest from Birmingham University, have shown a role for localised oestrogen in colon cancer for both men and women.

The fastest growing cancers in the Western world are prostate and skin cancer. Too often, and too glibly, the latter is attributed to white, defenceless people increasingly rushing off to the sunshine in the middle of winter. In fact such holidays have declined over the last couple of years, yet skin cancer rates have continued to increase. Could this not be due to the 'pre-sensitisation' of our skins by our increased 'oestrogen pools'? Certainly, melanoma has been shown to be oestrogen driven. Bizarrely, even some sunscreens contain toxic chemicals that mimic the action of oestrogen!

We do have government safe limits on these toxic chemicals. However they assume that the various chemical actions are not cumulative. Unfortunately, research by Dr Ana Soto has shown they are. Hungarian and Austrian researchers in 2003 showed much the same for toxic chemicals (like cleaners and bleaches) that could be breathed.

This info-book could be called 'Back to Basics'. For that is the real message. Find a company (at **icon** we recommend Neways, the only company endorsed by the US Cancer Prevention Coalition) that makes toxin-free products, keep clear of modern pesticides and herbicides, drink clean water, eat nourishing food sensibly and at all costs avoid synthetic oestrogen products like the pill and HRT. There is so much you can do to prevent or beat, if you already have, a hormonally driven cancer.

At **icon** a number of people ring us up to ask about their cancers. I always ask two questions up front:

1. Is your cancer hormonally driven?
2. What do you think caused your cancer?

Few people, apart from breast cancer sufferers, have

been told the answer to the first question by their doctors. Even fewer have stopped to think about the second question.

The fact is that most people, and their doctors, just don't think like this.

Sadly, whilst doctors are busy providing the orthodox expertise to try to rid their patients of the tumour, the oestrogen terrorist is still at work.

People who know me know I am most certainly not a 'doctor basher'. I think that anyone who spends seven years learning their profession and then dedicates their life to serving the lives of others deserves our utmost praise.

But the fact is that there is much you can do yourself to limit the terrorist in your body and many doctors simply do not know many of the proven biochemical facts behind oestrogen, which is undoubtedly and increasingly, **THE KILLER IN OUR MIDST**.

This book is meant to be very easy and quick to read, but to clearly cover exactly what action you can take to amplify your orthodox medical treatment.

Research shows that there is a tendency for some cancers (for example, prostate and breast) to 'run in the family'. If that is the case, the measures in this book will definitely help you stand a better chance of preventing the problem in the first place.

This book will also save me a lot of time. Hormonally

driven cancer is so common I have often had the same conversation five times in just a few hours!

Finally I'd like to thank Professor Trevor Powles, Dr John Lee, Dr Tessa Pollard, Dr Francisco Contreras, Dr Julian Kenyon, Dr Philippa Darbre, Sherrill Sellman, Professor Karol Sikora, Dr Rosy Daniel, and staff at The Haven in London who all indirectly and inadvertently helped provide me with research and ideas that I have used in this book! Plus of course Lindsey, Maggie, Melanie, Madeleine, Janet and Karen who read, commented on, and typed . . . and retyped!

Chris Woollams

1
WHAT ARE HORMONES AND WHAT'S THE PROBLEM?

Hormones are super-chemicals – the body's messengers. Even very small amounts of hormones have a monstrous effect on the actions of the human body.

Conventional theory runs that hormones are produced by your endocrine glands, for example – your pituitary, pineal gland, adrenal glands (kidneys), ovaries, thyroid, testes, etc.

These organs are directly under the command of the brain. This is most obvious when an animal is placed in a state of fear. When sensing danger the brain stimulates the production of adrenalin, the 'fight or flight' hormone, which prepares our whole body for action in dangerous circumstances.

Two facts about hormones are particularly relevant to the cancer issue:

Firstly, it is a little known fact **that every single cell in your body has the ability to produce localised hormones**. Back in 1982, John Vane won a knighthood, a Nobel Prize and a lot of money for his work on eicosanoids, hormones that last but a few seconds and are produced by the nuclear envelope in every cell in your body. The implications of this discovery are huge. For example, it is known that cortisol, the 'stress' hormone can stimulate the nuclear envelope at a localised level to produce 'bad' eicosanoids thus making the environment of that cell negative. In simple terms, what this means is: Get stressed and your breast cells or prostate cells get stressed too!! Steroids and insulin also have a similar, negative effect.

Secondly, in a healthy animal eating a natural toxin-free diet, drinking clean water and miles away from any harmful toxins and man-made carcinogens, the hormones are totally in balance within the body. This is called homeostasis.

However, when one single hormone is suddenly heightened or reduced, there is a knock-on effect to all the other hormones throughout the body. In the modern world much of the imbalance of hormones is caused either by our own actions, for example eating large carbohydrate-rich meals and stimulating the hormone insulin, or by third party toxins, for example the pesticide DDT, which has been proven to cause hormone imbalances and increase cancer risk. Both insulin and DDT are known to increase levels of oestrogen in the body.

2
SO CAN HORMONES CAUSE CANCER?

Well it is a fact that certain hormones have been specifically linked to increased cancer risk. But, given that all hormones interact (an excess of one causing an excess or a depletion of another) as I have said, changing the level of just one hormone, will alter the levels of all the others causing an imbalance and a toxic body, which will increase the risk of all manner of diseases including cancer.

For example, **melatonin** is a hormone produced about one and a half hours into sleep. It helps put you into a deeper sleep.

Studies in the USA (Harvard Medical School and Brigham) amongst night shift workers, and studies by SAS, the Scandinavian airline, on long-haul staff show that sleep deprivation or disruption causes a fall in melatonin levels and is associated with a higher risk of breast cancer in females. Harvard have gone on to look at nurses on night shifts and colon cancer and concluded that those with at least three night shifts a month for 15 years had a 35 per cent higher colon cancer risk.

Melatonin has well-established anti-carcinogenic properties and is itself an antioxidant. One of the actions of melatonin in the body is to neutralise free-radicals. These are the nasty, sticky molecules produced by, for example, smoking, drinking excess alcohol or eating saturated animal fats. Free-radicals like to rip pieces off passing molecules causing them to become equally sticky and prone to rip pieces off other molecules. When this happens to the cellular DNA, disaster strikes and a major step in the cancer process has taken place.

Professor David Spiegel of Stanford University Medical Centre in California, confirms that melatonin slows production of oestrogen adding that sleep protects against cancer, since oestrogen is known to proliferate cancer cells.

Cortisol is another hormone, dangerous in excess. In times of stress the brain sends messages to the adrenal glands and these are stimulated to produce more and more cortisol. As we saw in the last section, cortisol can actually change the localised environment of the cell and negatively affect its biochemical processes setting up the risk of a cancer cell forming.

3
WHAT EXACTLY IS
OESTROGEN?

Oestrogen is a naturally occurring human hormone. In fact it is not a single hormone, but a collective name for several variants. Oestradiol is the most potent, with oestrone and oestriol its much weaker sisters. All are secreted by the mammalian ovary. Men produce a little oestrogen too.

Five things are worth noting:

1. In the first half of her menstrual cycle, a woman's oestrogen levels build to the point of ovulation. Thereafter progesterone is the lead hormone, keeping oestrogen levels in check during the second half of the cycle.

2. Natural progesterone has the effect of balancing oestrogens in a normal healthy animal – female or male.

3. Natural progesterone is a precursor hormone – it can be converted naturally in the body into other essential steroid hormones, like testosterone or oestrogen. Wild yam is often considered a precursor to natural progesterone, but in fact it can be converted into any steroid hormone like testosterone or oestrogen.

4. Because this process involves an enzyme 'feed-back' system, when too much, say, oestrogen is produced the enzyme system cuts off production. Unfortunately there are many other providers of 'oestrogen' in the modern body which by-pass the system leaving oestrogen hopelessly swamping the progesterone.

5. Synthetic progesterone (e.g. Progestin) has no effect on this feedback system either. In fact synthetic progesterone has a number of negative side effects and it is linked to an increased risk of certain cancers.

The **importance** of considering **natural progesterone** every time you think or talk about oestrogen cannot be stressed enough. They are balancing twins in the natural state. It is a significant fact that women who have breast cancer operations in the second part of their cycle when progesterone is dominant have a 20 per cent greater chance of long-term survival. (i.e. it is safer to have a breast, oestrogen-dominated, cancer operation in the balancing part of the month.)

4
WHAT HAS OESTROGEN GOT TO DO WITH CANCER?

Every day, each of us produces 200–1000 pre-cancer cells as a result of our normal lives. Usually, our immune systems are more than capable of neutralising all of these. However, oestrogen acts as a helper, encouraging a cancer cell to spread its black messages to other healthy cells.

Oestrogen has a clear and special action in the cancer process. All cancer cells try to send out black messages to tell other healthy cells to turn rogue. Science is very clear on this. There are receptor sites on all healthy cells. Oestrogen molecules can 'combine' with messages from a rogue cancer cell plus a little carbohydrate and cause the rogue message to bind to these receptor sites on adjacent, but healthy, cells. This causes the healthy cell to turn 'rogue' too. And so single cancer cells can grow into a tumour or spread around the body via the blood or lymph systems.

The receptor sites work like the indentations on jigsaw puzzle pieces, and oestrogen helps the rogue cancer message fit.

Sadly, other synthetically produced molecules, which are not actually natural oestrogen but molecules that look fairly similar, can 'mimic' this action.

As Professor Trevor Powles of the Royal Marsden, Surrey, England, said recently in his interview with **icon**,

> "principally I think breast cancer has increased because of environmental reasons (including oestrogens and other agents/

chemicals in the food), and intake of hormones like HRT and oral contraceptives."

And he should know. He's the top man in the UK on breast cancer!

Secondly, oestrogen is known to 'starve' the power stations in healthy cells of oxygen (cancer cells have power stations that do not use oxygen). It alters the sodium/ potassium balance within cells, and if sodium displaces the power stations' potassium they become toxic, acid and inefficient. (See *The Tree of Life*, Chapter 3.) Starving cells of oxygen sets up conditions in which a cancer cell forms and thrives. Oestrogen can thus be both an initiator and a promoter of cancer.

An infamous anecdote concerns Dr Ana Soto of Tufts Cancer Centre in the USA who was growing cancer cells in a glass jar by stimulating them with oestrogen. When she blocked the oestrogen the cancer cells stopped growing. But suddenly after a considerable dormant period, even without added oestrogen, she noticed that they were growing again. Then she found that the glass jars had been replaced by plastic ones and the plastic was leaching oestrogen-like chemicals into her test cells.

Be warned. Your plastic packaging wrappers do this too, as do your plastic water bottles.

There are a whole host of ingredients in everyday toiletry and cosmetic products, in household products like bleaches, disinfectants and cleaners that once inside the bloodstream can mimic the action of oestrogen and help the rogue cancer develop into a tumour and pass its toxins on to other healthy cells.

Volatile organic carbon products may also be breathed in and have the same effect. Recently, Hungarian and Austrian scientists (**icon** September 2003) showed that these toxins collect at the crossroads in the air passages at 400 times the levels elsewhere.

Dr Ana Soto has also taken ten individual, everyday ingredients all at below government safe levels and injected them into animals, producing a full oestrogen response.

Both studies concluded that government safe levels of toxins needed to be seriously reviewed. What is clear is that our environments are adding to the oestrogen 'pool' in our bodies and this is causing more cancers. Cancer Research UK are quite clear on this and have concluded that we all have significantly higher oestrogen levels nowadays.

The ContamiNATION study by WWF found an average of 27 chemicals in the blood of the UK citizens tested, including PCBs and DDT. Dr Carol Rosenberg of Evanston-Northwestern Healthcare, USA published a study of 92,835 post-menopausal women in December 2003. In the study, 25 per cent of those who developed mild skin cancer went on to get a second different cancer, against a 'norm' of 11 per cent. Interestingly the skin cancers and the second cancers could all be counted as 'oestrogen driven'.

5
WHAT HAS OESTROGEN GOT TO DO WITH MEN AND THEIR CANCERS?

Men get prostate cancer. And they have melanoma, colon cancer and brain tumours too. Virtually all prostate cancers are thought to be hormonally responsive and caused largely by age related changes in the androgen/oestrogen balance. Many men with prostate cancer will have been advised that they have too much testosterone and this is the cause of their cancer. **This is actually misleading**. There is absolutely no scientific evidence that testosterone causes cancer of any sort. Nor is there any scientific evidence that testosterone **spreads** cancer. It may well be that many men who have prostate cancer also have high testosterone levels, just as they may have more dentures or thinning hair, but it is not the CAUSE nor the factor that SPREADS it.

The National Cancer Centre in Singapore have looked at factors that can stop the spread of prostate cancer, and they have shown that anti-oestrogens (e.g. ICI and Finasteride) both reduced spread and growth (by up to 50 per cent) of the prostate cells. This has been confirmed by Doctor Ian Thompson of the University of Texas. "Finasteride is the first drug that has been shown to reduce the risk of prostate cancer", he says. He believes that Finasteride slows or stops the conversion of 'harmless' testosterone into the real active problem, dihydrotestosterone (DHT), a very potent hormone. The conversion normally occurs due to oestrogen, indeed oestradiol.

Natural progesterone is another known 'limiter' of prostate growth and prostate cancer. Whilst synthetic progesterone is often given to prostate sufferers to curb their 'testosterone' levels, it will simultaneously inhibit their oestrogen levels too. So, this could well be a case of 'right drug – wrong reason!'

Not only is oestrogen a fundamental cause in the spread of cancers, research findings are clear that in men it is associated with a variety of factors from increasing prostate cancer risk to suppressing sperm levels (Handlesman et al; Concord Hospital, Sydney; March 2002). Indeed several studies have directly linked oestrogen mimics to declining sperm count. New research from the Monash Institute, Victoria, Australia (Risbridger, Bianco et al) has concluded that **prostate cancer is caused by localised production of oestrogens**. The research concludes that only androgen (e.g. testosterone) **combined with oestrogen** produces malignancy and that neither hormone alone is sufficient to produce it.

Oestrogen supplementation has even been tried as prostate therapy, but was withdrawn due to increases in blood clotting risk. The test drew no conclusions about the effect on the prostate cancers!

But at Hammersmith Hospital, London (April 2003) they have tested men with advanced prostate cancer and HRT patches and shown regression. This involved only 20 men over a short time scale and no comment was made whether the patches were oestrogen only or, as is more likely, whether this was a progesterone effect just that the aim was to shut off testosterone production!

Interestingly, research from the Wake Forest Cancer Institute, Carolina (published *BJC*, 13 October 2003) concludes that a gene CYP1B1 is linked to your susceptibility to prostate cancer. The gene has 13 variants and certain variants were found to respond to environmental toxins (oestrogen mimics).

The reason oestrogen is 'linked' to breast cancer so publicly and less to prostate, colon or melanoma is simply the volume of research being done on breast cancer compared with the others and the extra PR it all gets in the papers. But the fact is that **if oestradiol cannot be kept in check in males, prostate cancer is the risk**; just as oestrogen worsens the risk of cancers from colon to melanoma in **both** men and women.

This **mythology continues** when it comes to colon cancer and melanoma. Women on the pill have twice the risk of melanoma (Harvard Medical School, 1999). Colon cancer is caused by localised oestrogen (Birmingham University, 2000). Brain tumours linked to oestrogen toxins (NCI). In fact reading all the research findings (and I've read over 500 reports) I'm left with an impression that a lot of scientists take products like synthetic oestrogen or mixed synthetic oestrogen/progestin HRT and they try to 'build' their research around them in an attempt to find yet more possible uses.

Take for example some research by Boston University School of Medicine. In an interview about the findings, the lead researcher was saying that women with strong bones have lower breast cancer, and lower colon cancer. So if they could identify those with a hereditary risk of breast cancer and avoid giving them HRT, all others could benefit from HRT supplementation, as it strengthens bones and lowers colon cancer risk!

If this were true – and it doesn't appear to be, as we shall see – why do it? Oestrogen replacement is not the cure-all. It is actually dangerous.

In the West we consume the highest volumes of dairy in the world and have the highest blood calcium levels, but we have the lowest bone calcium levels because dairy depresses magnesium levels and the calcium cannot be taken up by bones without magnesium. Doctor Leo Galland of The Foundation for Integrated Medicine in the USA estimates that 40 per cent of people in the West are magnesium deficient. Exercise, particularly resistance training at any age, builds stronger bones and as we shall see, exercise actually reduces oestrogen levels in the body. So where is the hard evidence that HRT supplementation is the true answer? It's rather like taking two 'wrongs' and trying to make a 'right', as in the old saying, 'two wrongs don't make a right'.

Rather than oestrogen in HRT being a plus, epidemiology studies indicate **oestrogen actually contributes to colon cancer**, and localised oestrogen production may again be the key. So says M. English and team at the University of Birmingham and reported in August 2000 in *The British Journal of Cancer*.

Enzymatic action in the colon ordinarily converts oestradiol to the much weaker oestrone and this seems to be the protective driving force. If the enzymes don't do their job the oestradiol gets to work increasing colon cancer risk. Of course other factors are at play in colon cancer. High levels of fat consumption cause carcinogenic bile acids to be produced while fish oils, vitamins A and D have been shown to be protective – but that's another story.

The point is that far from being the 'linking bridge' as portrayed in Boston, the argument that HRT strengthens bones while strong bones are linked to people who have lowered levels of colon cancer, so therefore HRT helps protect in colon cancer, is a complete *non-sequitur*. An attempt to find use where none exists.

Let us look at another myth. Obviously the pre-dominant cause of melanoma is UV sunlight, this is a proven fact. Skin cancer is rapidly becoming the number two cancer in the UK. The reason given is our increasing desire to place our white bodies in tropical sunshine. However, studies have shown that sunscreens are only effective against UVB at 80 per cent levels, causing more concern.

But oestrogen levels can increase predisposition. One example of this is Harvard's findings using data from the Nurses Health Study (1976-1994). They found that those actually taking the oestrogen contraceptive pill had a doubled risk of melanoma. The findings are only true if the person is still taking the pill (*British Journal of*

Cancer November 1999). But the fact is that many things will give you higher levels of circulating oestrogen especially chemicals producing oestrogen mimics in both men and women. Worryingly, ingredients in sunscreens have been implicated in producing weak oestrogen mimic effects.

Feskanich et al (Department of Medicine, Harvard Medical School) have stated that 'oestrogens can increase melanocyte and melatonin count and cause hyper pigmentation of the skin.'

As we shall see later a number of xenoestrogens (oestrogen mimics) from a wide variety of everyday products will do this too.

Maybe, it's not just foreign holidays that are seeing the rise of skin cancer to become the second most common cancer in the UK.

Maybe oestrogen, and especially oestrogen mimics are at record levels in our bodies and predispose us to the adverse effects of sunlight.

6
SO, WHY MIGHT YOU HAVE EXCESS OESTROGEN?

Everyone of us has a 'pool' of oestrogen in our bodies. This pool in the twenty-first century is made up of our own natural oestrogen, natural oestrogens that we ingest (from foods, water, the pill etc.), and a variety of other chemicals that once in our bodies can 'mimic' the action of natural oestrogen, including synthetic oestrogen. So what are the specific reasons?

1. **You ingest more of it.**
   - oestrogens which are the animal's natural hormones come with all meats.
   - some animals have oestrogen and growth hormones added.
   - oestrogen can be found in recycled tap water.
   - the pill and HRT usually contain oestrogen.
   - alcohol consumption raises oestrogen levels.

2. **You make more of it yourself.**
   - fat consumption increases oestrogen production.
   - large carbohydrate-rich meals stimulate insulin production, which in turn stimulates oestrogen levels.
   - our own fat can increase our steroid levels and produce oestrogen; which is why fat people have more oestrogen in their bodies.

3. **You store it.**
   - fat is a wonderful solvent; if you are overweight you will store excess oestrogen that you should be excreting.
   - modern diets do not contain enough natural fibre to ensure excess oestrogen is properly excreted

4. **You are 'exposed' to synthetic oestrogen mimics, everywhere.**

   For example:
   - pesticides, e.g. DDT and Lindane.
   - industrial chemicals (from paints to detergents).
   - phthalates from plastics industry.
   - polychlorinated biphenyls (PCBs) e.g. used in electronics manufacturing.
   - volatile organic carbons (in glues, computer circuitry, bleaches, toiletries)
   - most perfume products.

Male or female, oestrogen and especially its synthetic mimics, are a modern hazard. Let us look at these reasons in more detail:

(A) YOU INGEST MORE OF IT

Compared to our ancestors, even just a few hundred years ago, we eat more meat. With the animal's protein and fat comes the animal's natural hormones (including oestrogen) plus any that may have been artificially added to help it grow.

Furthermore, with the animal's fat comes excess hormones like oestrogen, plus all the stored toxins and chemicals the animal has picked up from the pesticide and herbicide residues in the fields: plus the plethora of injections, antibiotics and growth enhancers (and even hormones) given to make it stronger, bigger and infection resistant.

Over 480 herbicides, pesticides and animal growth and 'protective' chemicals are legally permitted in farming in the USA, of which some two thirds have been shown to be directly or indirectly carcinogenic. 82 chemicals are legally permitted for animals alone. Britain is not far behind. And a large number of the pesticide residues, once they have entered our bodies, can 'mimic' oestrogen.

One infamous story of relevance concerned the pesticides DDT and Lindane in Israel. Extremely high levels of breast cancer were finally linked to these pesticides encroaching into the food chain. Dairy was identified as the main transporter. The pesticides were banned and over the following decade, cancer rates fell to more 'normal' levels.

The problem for you and I is that when Western Governments banned such infamous pesticides, they only banned their local use. The same companies still manufacture DDT but sell it abroad. Third World countries then grow their vegetables, use the pesticides and export the produce back to us!! Moreover, there are still many, many pesticides used in our countries whose effects are not fully known.

Synthetic oestrogen. When the contraceptive pill was first introduced there was only one study performed which could be called a proper clinical trial and that showed clear risks in taking it. Despite this a large dose oestrogen pill was launched for women. Fortunately, in the seventies and eighties levels of oestrogen were reduced as more links to cancer were found.

In 2002 Cancer Research UK figures showed the following increased risk of breast cancer for women taking oestrogen-based contraceptive pills.

Ever taken	**+ 26 per cent**
Taken into their 30s	**+ 58 per cent**
Taken into their 40s	**+ 144 per cent.**

The breast cancer rate in the UK is one in eight women. If a woman takes the pill in her forties, as over 10 per cent of the UK population does, the risk is estimated at one in three!

The Women's Health Initiative in the USA is a major study looking into a number of health issues. One part, where 16,000 healthy women aged between 50 and

79 were involved in a major clinical trial, the women using synthetic oestrogen and progesterone mixed HRT pills showed increases in breast cancer of 100 per cent plus increased rates of heart attacks, strokes and blood clots in the lungs. The trial was stopped 5.2 years into the 8 years for this combined pill, but still continues for the oestrogen-only pill where breast cancer increases were only around 27 per cent. (To put this figure in context, the increased risk of cancer, any cancer, attributed to smoking is 25 per cent, according to Sir Richard Doll and team in their pioneering work on tobacco.)

THE FDA HAS NOW INSISTED THAT ALL OESTROGEN CONTAINING PRODUCTS FOR POST-MENOPAUSAL WOMEN CONTAIN A HEALTH WARNING

– although they do this because of the heart risks not the cancer risks!

Cancer Research UK has recently found much the same in its 'Million Women' study – the leading synthetic oestrogen/progesterone brand doubled the risk of cancer, whilst oestrogen 'only' increases it 26 per cent. Findings also showed that HRT makes 'screening' less effective and breast cancer victims on HRT are 22 per cent more likely to die from disease.

But, in fact none of this is new. The Boston Nurses Questionnaire Study results were published almost ten years ago, says Sherrill Sellman, an expert in oestrogen, and followed 121,700 women for 18 years. Ten years of oestrogen alone showed the cancer risk rising by a third, whereas the mixed pill doubled risk.

Exactly the same findings.

The American Cancer Society in a study involving 240,000 post-menopausal women (1995), showed that the risk of fatal ovarian cancer was 40 per cent higher for women using the HRT pill for at least six years and 70 per cent higher after 11 years.

There is also evidence for girls in their formative years. Smoking during that time can increase breast cancer risk later in life by 70 per cent (Cancer Research UK); and Sellman confirms that the "earlier a girl goes on the pill the greater her eventual risk of contracting breast cancer, the larger her tumours and the worse her eventual prognosis." Sellman adds, "Oestrogen dominance actually accelerates the ageing process, increasing the risk of endometrial cancer and ovarian cancer, blood clots, strokes and high blood pressure."

Meanwhile 2.2 million women in the UK take HRT; a third over 50 presently take it, and half will take it at some time in their lives. The NHS dispensed 6 million prescriptions last year at a cost of £133 million.

Dutch doctors writing in the *Lancet* called on women taking HRT to stop immediately – whereas UK doctors told women to balance risks and benefits! However at the **icon** offices we rarely talk to women who know and understand the real risks. Wyeth, the company making a leading mixed hormone brand said, "These findings do not necessitate any urgent changes to treatment".

Do you feel that way too having read this?

Recycled water in cities is being found to contain increasing levels of oestrogens, thanks to users of HRT and the pill urinating into the system. Sadly there is insufficient attempt to clean the water of the hormones. Men and women have to understand this!

Lest you think this might be alarmist, work is being undertaken at the Athlone Institute of Technology, Ireland where a team of scientists are studying the effects of synthetic oestrogens in the sewage effluent and rivers, which is resulting in the feminization of male fish.

The American Chemical Society, has linked the widespread growth of oestrogen and its mimics to a decline in human male sperm count of 50 per cent over the last 50 years.

There can be little doubt that factors such as this are having a huge influence on levels of oestrogen in both men and women and their resulting cancers.

Of course, many people drink their water from plastic bottles, but phthalates (found in plastic and polyvinyl chloride containers) are also oestrogen mimics and leach into the water contained.

(B) YOU MAKE MORE OF IT

The World Health Organisation estimates that 70 per cent of all cancers have diet as a root cause.

Animal fat consumption stimulates oestrogen production. Research shows a 10 per cent increase in fat consumption increases female oestrogen levels by 20 per cent. Men who enjoy fried breakfasts have a three-fold increased risk of cancer over those who do not partake. Dr Tessa Pollard of Durham University made the front pages of British newspapers in September 2003, with the headline 'DIET CAUSES BREAST CANCER' and stated that "we tend to eat a lot of fatty food that increases steroid levels and oestrogen is a steroid." It is for the same reason that fat people tend to make more oestrogen for their own personal fat stores, and obesity is linked to a 20 per cent increase in, for example, breast cancer (NCI).

High calorie intake also stimulates oestrogen production. (Fat is, of course, high in calories.) The body's hormones work within a balanced system called homeostasis. Too much of one leads to imbalance with others being restricted, or over-produced.

An excess of insulin causes some hormones to be depleted whilst others – and notably oestrogen – are produced in larger quantities. Thus the typical Western eating pattern of two big meals a day leads to insulin, and oestrogen, surges. It is better to cut refined carbohydrate from the diet and 'graze' eating six small meals a day and thus controlling excesses of insulin.

Insulin is primarily produced in response to a diet high

in carbohydrates and sugars. Insulin prevents high blood sugar levels damaging the brain.

Separate research studies have shown that not just sugars and carbohydrate, but hydrogenated vegetable oils can cause pancreatic stress. A severely distressed pancreas can result in diabetes. Currently running at 8 per cent in American adults but a staggering 16 per cent in American children, poor diet is causing a serious, new epidemic. High sugar foods and drinks and fast foods with their hydrogenated vegetable oils pile up the negative pressure.

Pancreatic stress is not good news for cancer risk either. The pancreas is linked to the fundamental system of cellular control in the body and there is a strong school of thought that the pancreas has the ability to 'switch off' some cancer cells making them 'normal'. The fact is that a **5 per cent increase in calorie intake is associated with a 20 per cent increase in oestrogen levels, through the 'insulin link'**.

Interestingly, calorie restriction diets, such as those endemic to inhabitants of Okinawa, or wartime diets in Europe see an increase in health and longevity.

Another way (obviously unique to women) that oestrogen excesses are made, is the modern attitude to babies.

Diet primarily affects women's fertility. Women two hundred years ago were 'productive' normally from 16 to 38 years of age. They also had four to five children and breastfed them for at least a year and even two. Now the average New Yorker can have periods from age 12 to 52 and only one child, which she rarely breastfeeds for more than a few months, if at all. As a result her number of periods has doubled from 200 or so to 400. So, that's twice as many oestrogen surges by the time she reaches 50 as her ancestors were used to. Dr Pollard has shown that women in Mali, West Africa, have an average of 109 periods compared to a typical Western level of 400.

Cancer Research UK has confirmed that more babies, and breastfeeding longer can cut breast cancer rates. For every extra child there is a 7 per cent reduction; and a 6 per cent reduction for breastfeeding the child to month nine.

The Bush people in Australia or the Kalahari breastfeed their children until they are almost 5 years old in a toxin-free environment. They have no breast cancer.

Dairy is associated with a number of cancer risks. It is linked, for example, with reduced levels of vitamin D and zinc absorption (both critical, for example, in prostate cancer, while vitamin D is also deficient in colon cancers); and it also depresses the level of magnesium absorption, which is crucial to the proper working of every cell in your body. Poor magnesium levels are known to alter the biochemistry of the cell's mitochondria, or power stations. In cancer the power stations go drastically wrong using an oxygen-free energy system to promote rapid multiplication.

But dairy content can dramatically affect your oestrogen levels too:

◆ Its fat content brings with it a variety of toxins including oestrogen and oestrogen mimics as we saw above.

◆ Separate American, Swedish and Japanese research studies show that dairy can negatively affect your cells. Dairy, especially in the USA where growth hormones are used with cattle, contains Insulin-like Growth Factor (IGF1), which in the presence of milk protein more easily enters the human blood stream. Normally produced by the pituitary in very small amounts, IGF has been linked to changes in cellular metabolism, malignant cell proliferation and cancer in women and men (Cancer Prevention Coalition, Chicago and N.C.I.).

Swedish research announced in 1999, indicated **a direct link between the level of dairy consumed and a male's risk of prostate and testicular cancers!**

Professor Powles of the Royal Marsden stated a similar view in **icon** magazine recently. "I agree with Chris Woollams that there is a good argument in reducing animal fat intake" he says, "There is evidence that animal fat increases oestrogen levels and that that could be detrimental. We're trying to reduce oestrogen with a lot of treatments we're doing. Our general advice is to reduce animal fats and take unsaturated fats instead."

Another disrupting force is sodium. Sodium is ingested

as salt (sodium chloride) or as a meat preservative (sodium nitrite).

In every cell, in every body are little 'power stations' called mitochondria. Their energy production systems work using potassium and ideally in a slightly alkaline environment, which is created, in part, by the excesses of potassium over sodium inside the power stations.

High sodium levels in the body work their way into the cellular power stations displacing the potassium that normally makes the power stations run smoothly. The excess sodium makes the power stations more toxic and more acid and this environment inhibits some of the essential chemical reactions. It also blocks other systems where potassium was a necessary part of the equation.

As we have seen, our dairy-dominated diets depress magnesium. Magnesium works a little pump found in the cell wall. The job of this pump is to expel sodium and take in potassium so that our power stations can work properly and not become acid and toxic and potentially cancerous.

Finally, sodium is a serious endocrine disrupter and significantly inhibits the production and the action of certain hormones.

And as we have said, if one hormone goes out they all go out, making your body toxic and cancer more likely.

WE ALL EAT TOO MUCH SODIUM . . .

Sausages, bacon, crisps, peanuts, fast food, processed foods, dried meats like hams and salami: Do you recognise the diet??

Four slices of white or malted bread, three bags of crisps or three bowls of breakfast cereal each provide 1 gram of sodium!

The average American eats a massive 12 gms per day of sodium, the average Brit about 10 gms. The FSA in the UK has decreed a safe level of 6 gms for adults and 3 gms for children. In the wild, as an animal thousands of years ago, you were unlikely to have eaten any at all. So much so that salt licks needed to be found; and in the middle ages salt was a form of currency, because of its scarcity. It was an important currency in bartering and is the origin of the word salary. I feel strongly that a level of 1 to 2 gms per day is ample, and this is the figure decreed by the US Institute of Medicine in February 2004.

. . . AND NOT ENOUGH
POTASSIUM AND MAGNESIUM

High potassium and high magnesium foods include pulses, like lentils, chickpeas, broad beans, peas, kidney beans etc, nuts, brown whole rice, bananas, apples, green leafy vegetables, and jacket potatoes.

You should eat five times more potassium a day than sodium to ensure your cells and your hormones stay healthy and balanced.

Oestrogen causes sodium to flood into the cell and render it less efficient, more acid and more toxic. As the cells' power stations become more toxic, the nature of the chemical reactions changes and they use less and less oxygen. A power station that works without oxygen is a cancer cell power station. Again high oestrogen lowers cellular oxygen levels.

Finally alcohol intake stimulates oestrogen production for women and men. Cancer Research UK showed one extra glass of wine per day raised breast cancer risk by 6 per cent.

(C) YOU STORE MORE OF IT

Overweight people have a 20 to 60 per cent higher risk of cancer, depending upon which research study you read. For example, the National Cancer Institute in the USA found in 2003 that obesity is linked to a 20 per cent increase in cancer risk (by comparison, smoking increases it 25 per cent). In particular, significant rises of oestradiol in the body were linked to obesity.

Erasmus College, Rotterdam reanalysed 70 years of USA population data and showed that women and men who were 4 kgs overweight lost 3 years from their life expectancy; if the excess was 10 kgs, men lost 5.8 years and women 7 years.

Fat is a wonderful solvent and it will dissolve all manner of toxins and hormones you would ordinarily want to excrete from your body for safety's sake.

Of course oestrogen (and oestrogen mimics) are one of the main toxins stored. If you carry fat round your stomach, think seriously about your personal 'toxic waist'.

Be warned.

Oestrogen mimics are highly soluble in fat.

(D) YOU ARE SURROUNDED BY IT!

Chemicals with the ability to become synthetic oestrogen mimics once they enter our blood streams surround us all.

Volatile organic carbons (VOCs) and harmful chemicals are given off readily by a number of everyday substances. For example, petrol fumes when filling your car; glues used to attach floor or ceiling tiles or to stick together cheaper wood products; inks used by faxes, gases from the circuitry of computers; gases from bleaches and all manner of household cleaners and disinfectants, dry cleaning and chlorine products. Most paper products are treated with chlorine. Toxins linked to cancer abound in our everyday lives. Carpets hold and encourage air dust and so the gases join with the dust particles and are inhaled.

Cosmetics and toiletries, especially perfumed products are a Pandora's box of oestrogen mimics. Their ability to be absorbed by the skin into the blood stream is worsened by chemicals such as sodium lauryl sulphate (SLS), present in most soap, shampoos and toothpastes. SLS weakens the impermeability of the skin by 40 per cent allowing more toxins to cross its supposed barrier effect. Indeed, all modern research proves that your skin is a carrier not a barrier. In the **Appendix**, I include a full list of **toxins in everyday toiletries** and an article reproduced from **icon** magazine on **Toxins in the Home**.

But, of course, men are not immune. They wash their faces, clean their teeth, use perfumed shaving foam, aftershave and body sprays.

They sit in poorly ventilated rooms with computers and faxes and they drink their coffee made from recycled tap water.

The biggest worry is that there is a strong correlation between oestrogen mimics and the induction of genotoxicity. 90 per cent of all such mutations are carcinogenic.

Worse, oestrogen mimics are widely diverse and it is, frankly, hard to test all of them. Worse still, many of them only form once inside the body, and worst of all, these effects have been found to be cumulative. David Feldman, Professor at Stanford University said, "The cumulative effect of xenoestrogens may be much greater than any individual molecule". Now this fear has been clearly established as truth by Dr Anna Soto of Tufts Cancer Research Center in the USA in her research.

Oestrogen mimics build up in the bodies of each of us and their effects are proven to be cumulative.

Recently The Royal Commission reported in the UK on toxins in the home and environment, confirming the case that the Cancer Prevention Coalition (run by

Professor Samuel Epstein of Chicago University) has been saying for years. Levels of such toxins permitted need to be greatly revised downwards; indeed much work is still needed to identify them in the first place! Imagine all the toxins in the thousands of toiletry, cosmetic and household ingredients used every day. Arguably, many ingredients are toxic and a great number are carcinogens or xenoestrogens. But to research them all is going to take decades and changing safe limits or banning them all would have huge implications for industry and the economy and so is unlikely to happen. Vote with your wallet and seek out toxin-free suppliers like Neways, for example, who make a whole range of products from lipsticks to baby products and shampoos to washing up liquids. All without the use of any of the feared toxins listed in the Appendix.

(E) YOU ARE BEING
ENCOURAGED TO USE IT!!

Mythology abounds to the point of downright mis-information. All the scientific indications are that we all have far, far more oestrogen in our bodies than nature intended. Yet doctors seem to want to give us more of it. For example, HRT is given supposedly because oestrogen levels fall dramatically at the menopause. But since they start in modern women at far higher levels than were present in her ancestors, where is the evidence that they have fallen too low and need supplementing with synthetic oestrogen? Indeed, natural oestrogen levels only fall to about 60 per cent of 'normal' – just enough to prevent ovulation. Whereas progesterone falls completely, with about 3 per cent of original levels being produced by the adrenal glands. In men several studies seem to indicate that our oestrogen pool (of hormones and mimics) simply slowly grows as we age!

Osteoporosis? No, that is in part due to excesses of dairy, a lack of load-bearing exercise (which is why men are now getting it more frequently) and stress which causes bones to leach calcium. Over use of steroids is another cause, as are excess caffeine and sodium both of which leach calcium from the bones. But in the West we have the highest levels of circulating blood calcium and the lowest levels in our bones. Why? Because you need magnesium to get it into the bones and dairy suppresses magnesium. Catch twenty two. Vitamin D will also help assimilation (sunshine and fish are the best sources).

Hot flushes and night sweats? Research shows these can be corrected with natural progesterone just as effectively as synthetic oestrogen.

In fact, all the indicators are that women in the West have much higher levels of oestrogen in their blood streams than women in the East even after the menopause. The same applies to men. And cancer rates are far, far lower historically in the East and more primitive countries. Dr Pollard has been taking evidence worldwide and proving exactly this point.

Sadly the reason synthetic oestrogen is recommended like 'sweeties' is that day in, day out usage is big business. Very big business.

Natural progesterone can be processed from inexpensive herbs and cannot be patented, so no companies will get rich from it. Worse, synthetic progesterone (Progestin, for example) has a history of side effects – for example, its cancer risks in combined HRT pills or as a probable cause of certain cancers in humans. Some doctors even get confused between the names Progestin and progesterone, thinking that all such progesterone is tarnished by the HRT research findings. As a result of all this doctors dish out the synthetic oestrogen and progesterone and ignore the natural progesterone.

(F) THE DOUBLE WHAMMY

(AT THE MOMENT WHEN THERE ARE MORE TOXINS AROUND TO CAUSE MORE PROBLEMS THAN EVER BEFORE, WE HAVE THE WEAKEST EVER IMMUNE SYSTEMS)

Professor Karol Sikora, former head of the World Health Organisation's cancer programme, in his speech 'The future of cancer care', claimed that of the 10 million new cancers worldwide each year, 3 million are due to dietary inadequacies, 3 million due to toxins and pollution, and 1.5 million are due to infection (e.g. viral). He further believes that cancer treatments in the UK pay **no attention** to these factors – and he is right.

Cancer is a multi-step process; one report said it took six steps to turn a normal cell into a rogue cell. Some factors e.g. asbestos or talcum powder can apparently short-circuit all the steps of cancer production. (Talc, asbestos-like in its formula, has been linked to ovarian cancer).

As we said, even a normal healthy individual produces 200–1000 'cancer' cells per day. But a normal healthy individual has a strong immune system that identifies and neutralises them. So it follows that to avoid cancer, one essential is simply 'Love your immune system'. **American research has shown that people with weak immune systems get more cancers.**

But whilst there are more toxins around, we have weakened immune systems less able to deal with them. If, for example, you have a poor diet with limitations on vitamin and mineral consumption, you expose your body to dangers.

At the **icon** offices, our observation is that the great majority of newly diagnosed cancer patients are **nutritionally toxic** (for example, from too much salt, junk food, processed food, lack of vegetables and fruit etc) and/or **nutritionally deficient**. The latter has been borne out by the French Su Vi Max study published in Autumn 2003. 17,000 adults between 35 and 60 years of age were given an anti-oxidant supplement containing beta-carotene, vitamin E, vitamin C, selenium and zinc. In seven years this resulted in a 31 per cent decline in male cancers and, crucially, a 37 per cent decline in cancer mortality for both men and women.

One of the principal nutrient and toxic dangers is attack from **yeasts**, **viruses** or **parasites**. A weakened immune system can allow a virus to take hold. Professor Robert Souhami, Director of Clinical Research for Cancer Research UK, says: "Around 15–20 per cent of all cancers are caused by viruses, so it's vital that we get a better handle on the role of viral infection." For example, some **breast cancer** patients (perhaps only 1–2 per cent) have been found to have the **shingles** virus. About the same proportion of **prostate patients** have been found to have the **herpes** virus.

In fact these figures could be a vast underestimate. The role of viruses in research was studied until 30 years ago then dropped. Now with better equipment reports from the USA on mouse viruses and breast cancer, or virus studies in Australia, suggest 40 per cent of cancer may be viral.

Cervical cancers have been linked to the Human Papillomavirus. **Ovarian** cancer may be triggered by chlamydia.

But there are many 'types' of parasite. Yeasts are, in fact, the most common invader of both men and women.

USA and UK cancer clinics I have visited feel that **every** cancer patient has a parasite of some sort – most usually a yeast/*candida albicans* infection. And their growth and effects in our bodies are worsened by steroids, antibiotics and chemotherapy, so much so that in 1993 the American Oncology Review reported that the majority of patients who died after chemotherapy in fact **succumbed to the effects of candida and not the cancer!!!!**

But the overall point is that poor diet, for example, is linked to a reduction of the immune system and that allows other factors to exploit and further add to the weakness.

Furthermore, many factors in the products we use are working to weaken the immune system further. For example from the CPC Chicago, Athlone Institute of Technology, Ireland, NCI in the USA:

Excess oestrogen and especially pesticides and toxic oestrogen mimics have been clearly shown to weaken the immune system.

Oestrogen mimics have also been shown to deplete folic acid, which is essential to proper DNA replication, an essential in preventing cancer (Yuriy Burkin, Professor NICR Moscow).

Finally, **oestrogen mimics are known endocrine disrupters** (Athlone Institute of Technology, Ireland). As such, they disrupt the proper balance and function of all your hormones. But certain hormones are a crucial part of your cancer-cell-attacking immune defence and to disrupt them is to expose you to an increased risk of cancer.

As a little example, nail polishes and cleaners have toxic ingredients and your brain can accumulate them as it is very fatty. Girls in nail salons in the USA have eight times the levels of brain tumours than are found in normal adults.

(G) PLANT OESTROGENS:
HELP OR HINDRANCE?

Simultaneously, we have rejected the foods that protected us. The wealth of natural foods like fruit and vegetables, freshly picked and in season, is being replaced by packaged foods, fast foods, refined foods and a host of other nutritionally deficient and sometimes downright toxic foods.

Food picked unripe and brought half way across the world must be expected to be nutritionally deficient. Kirlian photographs show they are energy deficient. And the only place a fruit can ripen is on the vine not in a shop-keeper's window. Ripening is the time when vitamins and minerals are assimilated. Food 'faddism' is proving poor nourishment. Back in 1906 Sajan Ishazuka, the founder of macrobiotics, told us to eat: "Fresh, locally grown and in season fruits and vegetables". Only in this way can we hope to ingest their full protective benefits.

Refining is another nutritionally deficient exercise. Refined wheat, for example in pasta, has lost 80–90 per cent of its vitamins and minerals, 99 per cent of its fibre and yet its calorie per gm figure has increased by 7–10 per cent.

Far, far more on this subject can be found in *The Tree of Life*, my book totally devoted to understanding what foods we need to **add** back into our diets in order to fully protect ourselves.

The one food group that is most relevant to the oestrogen issue is those containing **phytoestrogens or isoflavones**. These are found in **many vegetables and fruit**, but particularly in **beans and pulses**.

Back in 1900, 30 per cent of our protein came from this group of natural protectors. Now it is only 2 per cent in the modern Western world. This shows how animal protein (and with it, fat) has encroached into our diet.

But it also shows how we have lost powerful protectors – beans and pulses were actually giving us all, men and women, protection from oestrogen excesses.

Beans and pulses contain isoflavones or phytoestrogens. Phytoestrogens are plant oestrogens, much weaker (about 60 per cent) than human oestrogen and with a slightly different chemical formula. However, the body's systems recognise their presence and produce less human oestrogen to compensate. Phytoestrogens have thus had a vital regulatory role in our evolution.

We have lost that role and with it the protection.

Phytoestrogens also have the ability to join with carbohydrate and sit on, and block, healthy cellular receptor sites, the very ones that oestrogen helps the cancer message attack. So this is a second way phytoestrogens keep human oestrogen in check.

In the East the most discussed source of phytoestrogens is soya, although the Far Eastern diet contains such high levels of plants and vegetables that women in parts of China can have phytoestrogen levels 1000 times higher than found in the blood of women living in New York.

The West's phytoestrogens were commonly found in lentils, chickpeas, beans, peas, kidney beans, flageolet and all pulses – foods we just do not eat any more, although pulses are still common in the 'Mediterranean Diet', which is renowned for being more protective against cancer despite its high fat levels.

Even Hippocrates regularly used the herb red clover, which is currently being studied with breast cancer patients at the Royal Marsden.

Red clover has a long history of use as a medicinal herb. It is an excellent blood purifier that over time gradually cleanses the bloodstream and corrects deficiencies in the circulatory system. But among classic herbalists, it is probably best known as a herb for treating cancer and is found as a central ingredient in a number of herbal anti-cancer formulas, including the Hoxsey formula, Jason Winter's tea and Essiac tea.

Researchers at the National Cancer Institute have confirmed that there are indeed anti-tumour properties in red clover. One, genistein, has the ability to prevent tumours from developing the blood supplies they need to survive, thus starving them and killing them. Genistein is the same biochemical considered to be the main beneficial ingredient in soya. But red clover has a significant advantage over soya, as it contains about ten times the level found in soya of all four main oestrogen isoflavones, including daidzein and genistein. In addition to isoflavones, red clover contains another class of anti-cancer phytoestrogen compounds called coumestans, for example, biochanin and formononetin. Consuming red clover isoflavones results in higher blood levels of daidzein and genistein, moderate blood levels of biochanin, and low levels of formononetin. Soya consumption does not result in any increase in biochanin or formononetin in the blood.

Trinovin from red clover actually contains four isoflavones and may have some effect on prostate cancer in tests reported in *Cancer Epidemiology Biomarkers and Prevention* Vol. 11, December 2002. In a proportion of the sample tested there were clear improvements in the disease.

Early in 2004 Professor Trevor Powles is expecting the results on a trial at the Royal Marsden that has been going for two years, where 400 women who don't have breast cancer have been given genistein. (Genistein is used by some doctors and nutritionists like Professor Lawrence Plaskett, Vice Chairman of The Nutritional Cancer Therapy Trust, in the treatment of hormonally driven cancers.)

> "We're just starting to do the analysis now, . . . We're looking at all the potential effects on bone, breasts and hormone levels with naturally occurring sugars like genistein – from soya and red clover – which are phytoestrogens (naturally occurring oestrogens or anti-oestrogens). If the results are negative, it doesn't mean that red clover doesn't work. We might have got the

wrong phytoestrogen mix, or wrong dose, so we will do further trials because I'm sure that there will be natural products that will be very beneficial. I think they will help because in Chinese/Far Eastern diets, where these levels are high, breast cancer incidence is low and the level of osteoporosis is low. So there's something in those diets that's protecting people against both diseases."

Cancer Research UK conducted research with women in Singapore and showed those with the highest levels of genistein in their bloodstreams had the lowest levels of breast cancer. Similar research in China applied to men and prostate cancer.

You may read some criticism of soya but you must separate this from the biochemical action of the phytoestrogens. Soya is relatively new to the West – it arrived in the sixties. As a result it can cause allergies. It also has quite high fat content and, as such, was not favoured in the extreme anti-cancer diet of Dr Gerson (nor was any fat!). His daughter Charlotte correctly notes that all pulses contain phytic acid, which inhibits mineral absorption in the gut. Frankly, this is not a problem unless you are on an extreme cancer-busting diet. Finally soya, like all pulses, is an incomplete protein (for example, it lacks vitamin B12). Soya therefore should be used in a limited way in your diet.

Citrus phytoestrogen (isoflavones) has also had some limited success with the treatment of brain tumours.

RECENT SCIENTIFIC RESEARCH COVERED IN icon MAGAZINE

The volume of research concerning oestrogen and its mimics is overwhelming. Here is a summary of the latest featured **in just the last three months in icon**!

◆ Swedish research results in 2003 showed that two thirds of a list of perfumed products, ranging from perfumes themselves, to shampoos, deodorants, body sprays and hair colourings contained chemicals that, once inside the blood stream, were oestrogen mimics. One in particular DEHP, when found in pregnant women is known to cause genital abnormalities in their unborn male offspring – including higher rates of testicular cancer

◆ Ana Soto of Tufts Cancer Research Center (USA) took ten different oestrogen mimics all at Government permitted 'safe levels' and, in her animal experiments, witnessed an full oestrogen response, concluding that the effects had to be cumulative.

◆ Hungarian and Austrian scientists (*Journal of Applied Physiology*) have shown that inhaled pesticides collect at certain 'junctions' in the lungs. The reasons are not fully understood but the levels are

400 times higher there than normal. Again, this accumulation necessitates a rethink on permitted toxin levels by governments

♦ USA research shows that women who use considerably more products (face creams, lipsticks, eye shadows, hair dyes, cleansers etc, etc.) than their men, have four times the level of such toxins in their bloodstreams.

♦ Dr Philippa Darbre (Cancer Research, Reading University) has linked breast cancer in men and women to antiperspirants (*Journal of Applied Toxicology*).

♦ USA research showed that women with breast cancer were five times more likely to have DDT residues and nine times more likely to have HCB residues in their blood as had the control sample of 'normal' women.

♦ Women who are full-time housewives, or women who work from home have 40 per cent more toxins in their bloodstreams than women who go out to work.

♦ *International Journal of Cancer* reported links between dark hair dyes and cancer.

♦ EU bans 80 garden sprays – weed killers and pesticides. Disposal of these toxins is a real problem; must not be poured down sink or into drains.

◆ Euro MP says, "Government legislation needed": under-sink products such as washing powders, stain removers and detergents – potential health hazards and little information available.

◆ The findings of a Royal Commission, set up in the UK by The Queen and Prime Minister, concluded that only a fraction of the industrially produced chemicals have been studied in any depth and their chemical interaction effects were unknown. More work was recommended. Subsequently, the Commission found the Government's response to their study 'weak'.

◆ The ContamiNATION study by WWF in Britain looked at 77 dangerous chemicals in human blood finding 27 on average, and 45 in one person. These included pesticides like DDT and Lindane, PCBs and PCDEs (fire retardants). Worse, mums can pass them on to their babies by breastfeeding.

7
OK, I UNDERSTAND THE PROBLEM. WHAT'S THE SOLUTION?

SOLUTION CHECKLIST

Firstly let us summarise the broad areas of the solution:

1 Make less oestrogen:

- cut down on animal fats and fats in general
- cut out all dairy products
- buy organic food from a known supplier to limit consumption of herbicides and pesticides and other toxins.
- cut empty calories and hydrogenated vegetable oils; eat 5–6 small meals a day and no refined carbohydrates.
- ensure a 'clean' supply of water, e.g. use a reverse osmosis filter.
- have more babies and breastfeed them longer!

2 Eat more 'protective' foods, like phytoestrogens

3 Build your natural progesterone

- and cut synthetic oestrogen (and progesterone) supplements.

4 Cut oestrogen mimics from your everyday lives:

- household toxins, for example, cosmetics and toiletries toxins and perfumes.

Before we look at the 'solution checklist' in more detail let us summarise some of the simple myths doctors live with and that we have mentioned so far, by referring to the accurate biochemistry of the hormones oestrogen and progesterone.

1. Doctors measure oestrogen levels by taking blood tests. **This is wrong**. The only accurate measurement is to take saliva tests. A blood test will not just measure free oestrogen, but also protein-bound (non-bioavailable) oestrogen. Worse, blood tests measure plasma or serum levels. But most of the free oestrogen is carried by the red blood cells and escapes measurement. The tests doctors do are inaccurate. **Only a saliva test is accurate**. (Cummings et al *NEJM* September 1998).

2. Not only is a blood test of oestrogen inaccurate but the whole idea of measuring oestrogen on its own is absolutely irrelevant. The only relevant measurement of oestrogen is its level relative to progesterone since, in their natural state, they are mutually balancing.

3. For women, conventional medicine will tell you that at menopause your 'symptoms' (hot flushes, osteoporosis, heart attack risk) are brought on by the sudden fall of oestrogen. In fact **this is simply not true**. Your oestrogen level gradually declines over the decade before the menopause.

   Secondly, the implication is that oestrogen levels have suddenly declined to zero. In fact, **oestrone**

falls only about 40 per cent, and oestradiol about 60 per cent during this time. So by no means is this decline 'total', or even near total. There easily remains enough 'oestrogen' to keep all bodily functions intact save for egg production and pregnancy.

However, at the same time a hormone (the sex hormone binding protein, SHBC) has grown in volume and this blocks the action of the remaining oestrogen causing some of the post-menopausal symptoms. This blocking hormone can be neutralised by natural progesterone.

4. However progesterone has declined severely in the decade before menopause to almost zero levels. A little – about 3 per cent of original levels – is produced by the adrenal glands.

5. A healthy ratio of progesterone to oestradiol (in accurate saliva tests) is 200:1 to 300:1. However after menopause this ratio is greatly **exceeded**. The only way to restore the balance is to prescribe natural progesterone (or cause a further and possibly unnatural decline in oestrogen). Even in men this is the case, where oestradiol far outweighs progesterone levels after menopause. Only recently has the medical profession even contemplated that men might have a menopause.

6. Synthetic progesterone cannot replicate the effects of natural progesterone in this equation; natural progesterone is a precursor for and regulator of,

hormones like oestrogen and testosterone through a natural enzymatic feedback system. Synthetic progesterone has no influence on this but does have some serious side effects. For example, it increases the risk of coronary problems while natural progesterone prevents them. Furthermore, synthetic progesterone seems to block many androgen receptors and therefore the action of a number of important hormones.

As Dr Contreras, one of the top integrated cancer doctors in the World and head of The Oasis of Hope Hospital, Mexico said to me, the issue with hormonally driven cancers is simple. "Cut the oestrogen." This strategy is confirmed by leaders of the orthodox medical world too like Professor Trevor Powles. Even the new female 'wonder drug' Armidex (or Anastrozole) which is aimed at post-menopausal wowen at risk of breast cancer works simply by 'cutting these women's high levels of oestrogen'. Anybody who has studied the detailed biochemistry of these hormones knows this to be the true solution. There are a number of ways of doing this as we shall now list. One way is to increase the levels of natural progesterone in the body.

The science of oestrogen and the balancing natural progesterone is also detailed by experts such as the late Dr John Lee and Sherrill Sellman who have spent long periods of research on the subject. Their conclusions are well documented and clear, with supporting scientific evidence.

The first conclusion then for hormonally driven cancers, from prostate to breast, is to avoid giving yourself yet more oestrogen.

At **icon** we are clear on this – for example, we have talked to a large number of women who went on to HRT in the previous year and now have cancer. Our belief is that the problem was already building for these people – the extra oestrogen in HRT merely tipped them over the edge. So:

Come off the pill,

come off HRT.

Now.

The second conclusion is to avoid ingesting or making more oestrogen through poor dietary choices:

◆ Change your eating habits and pay serious attention to controlling your weight.

◆ Ideally eat 5 per cent less calories per day than you need.

◆ Eat five to six small meals per day not two big ones. Avoid fried food and fried breakfasts. Eat more natural fibre in vegetables, fruits and whole/complete grains.

◆ Avoid high glycaemic index foods – e.g. refined wheat products (pasta, pizza, bread), refined grains in general, sugars, fizzy soft drinks and empty calorie drinks, alcohol and fast and processed foods.

◆ Avoid salt (especially in dried meats, crisps, peanuts, sausages, bacon, processed foods, tinned foods, mass market bread and breakfast cereals).

◆ Eat more potassium, magnesium and phytoestrogen rich foods, like pulses, nuts and fruits and green vegetables.

◆ Avoid saturated and polyunsaturated fats, concentrate on monounsaturated fats (like olive oil, nuts, seeds).

◆ Avoid recycled tap water. Avoid plastic bottled drinks. Use a distillation system or a reverse osmosis water filter (probably the best route to take as then you can drink it hot or cold, and cook in it too).

◆ Avoid dairy and replace with a **little** soya and/or rice milk.

◆ Go organic – meat, vegetables, fruit.

◆ Increase intake of indole-3-carbinol foods like broccoli, brussel sprouts, kale and green leaf vegetables. (*The Journal of Biological Chemistry*, 6 June 2003 – I3C is a potent suppressor of prostate cancer cell spread and is also effective with other hormonal cancers like breast and endometrial cancer).

The third conclusion is to take supplements to boost your weakened immune system.

For example –

A good colloidal multivitamin and mineral, for example, Neways Maximol	(as directed on bottle)
Beta-carotene	(3 x 6 mgs during day)*
Vitamin C	(1 gm time release per day)
Vitamin E	(400 IUs per day)
Zinc	(15–25 mgs per day)
Selenium	(200 micrograms per day)
Lycopene	(25 mgs per day)
B complex with 0.3 mgs of Biotin, 400 micrograms folic acid and choline and inositol	(1 tablet per day)
Pure Cod Liver Oil	(500 mgs per day)
Astragalus	(as directed on bottle)
Echinacea	(as directed on bottle)
Cat's Claw	(as directed on bottle)

Also helpful in hormonally driven cancers are both soya and citrus isoflavones and bioflavenoids.

*N.B. Beta-carotene is a fragile vitamin, easily attacked by free radicals and destroyed by saturated and polyunsaturated fats. It works best when in combination with other anti-oxidants which act to protect it. We find that Neways Revenol, with its high levels of antioxidants takes this fragility into account and is first class.

The fourth conclusion is to lose your fat. Take, ideally daily, exercise. This could be via a gym or, less strenuously, yoga or Tai Chi.

◆ Exercise helps balance your hormones and it helps beat depression and stress.

Dr George Brainard and his research team at the Centre of Integrative Medicine of Thomas Jefferson University in Philadelphia tested the cortisol levels of yoga novices before and after a 50 minute session and showed levels decreased far more after just one session of yoga, even if it was the participant's first ever session, than during periods of rest. (Doctors would normally tell stressed people to rest.) Cortisol, the stress hormone, is known to suppress the immune system, constrict blood vessels and alter negatively the immediate environment of all cells in the body. It is implicated in cancer. Other research has shown that its negative effects can be limited to some degree by fish oils (omega 3), aspirin, garlic and ginger.

'Happy' hormones (endorphins) are also released during aerobic exercise and these can balance adrenalin and other negative hormones.

Resistance training increases levels of human growth hormone in the body. Hgh is known to reduce fat levels in the body and act as a free-radical neutraliser.

◆ Exercise helps get oxygen into your bloodstream and tissues. Oxygen actually kills cancer cells.

Otto Warburg won a Nobel Prize for showing this fact. Oxygen levels are also linked to depression and vice versa – the more oxygen in your blood the less depression.

◆ Exercise helps you breathe fully and properly and helps you expel toxins through the lungs and pores.

◆ Exercise helps you control your weight.

Perhaps the particular finding of most relevance is the most recent. In September 2003, *The Journal of the American Medical Association* reported that women who engaged in 1.25 to 2.5 hours of moderate exercise weekly had an 18 per cent lower risk of breast cancer. Lead researcher Dr Anne McTiernan of the Fred Hutchinson Cancer Research Seattle says the exercise need not be super strenuous. The Center for Disease Control and Prevention in the USA recommends 30 minutes **daily** exercise and the findings suggest that moderate exercise clearly reduces oestrogen levels.

◆ Exercise helps you **lose your fat**, and your fat makes and stores oestrogen you do not need.

The fifth conclusion is to quit smoking, to avoid passive smoking and to moderate alcohol consumption.

Smoking, including passive smoking, increases risk of all cancers in the body, not just lung cancer. Tobacco smoke is twice as dangerous for women than men because of genetic factors in airways, carried uniquely on the X chromosome – and women have two X chromosomes, men only one.

Cancer Research UK have proven that every extra regular glass of alcohol increases breast cancer risk 6 per cent.

Conclusion six is to visit a good homeopath and ask to be tested for yeast and other parasite infections.

He will be able to test you using the BEST or VEGA systems. And he should be able to advise you on how to get rid of them, should they be present. Taking an acidophilus supplement is a good idea anyway. Natural products like wormwood, caprylic acid, garlic, Pau d'Arco, neem, clove, black walnut, fennel and slippery elm can all help. Americans are much more conscious of the likelihood of having a parasite than we are in the UK and they will often be checked every 6 months or so. In the UK it is simply ignored, which is curious to say the least. 70 per cent of British people have a yeast infection – typically thrush in women, or yellow toe nails in men are sure signs. Meanwhile liver fluke have quadrupled in our livestock since 1997 according to Government data.

Both the BEST and VEGA systems will also be able to tell if you have high levels of toxins or, for example, heavy metals in your body.

The seventh conclusion is to talk to an integrated medical practitioner about taking natural, herbal progesterone.

Unlike oestrogen which is a family of hormones each with a slightly different action, progesterone is just a single hormone. It is produced by the ovaries, the testes and the adrenal glands. In men and women after menopause it is totally overwhelmed by the body's oestrogen pool.

Sherrill Sellman's view is that "Natural progesterone should oust oestrogen from centre stage." And that is definitely true. In men, if natural progesterone could balance the high oestrogen levels, prostate cancer risk would be reduced.

A study at John Hopkins in Baltimore and reported in *The American Journal of Epidemiology* showed conclusively that women with lowered progesterone have a five and a half-fold increased risk of breast cancer and a ten-fold increased risk of any cancer.

Less effective is wild yam as supplement or cream. This helps to stimulate the adrenal glands, the only internal source of natural progesterone after the menopause – female or male. But wild yam is merely a precursor ingredient for hormones like progesterone, oestrogen and testosterone.

Finally, conclusion and action point 8 is:

Find a provider of toiletry and make-up products, soaps, detergents, disinfectants and cleaning products that are completely non-toxic.

Our recommendation, like that of CPC, is Neways, but it would be ideal if more manufacturers took these challenges seriously across their whole range of toiletries, cosmetics, bathroom and household products.

The Hour Glass

When people with cancer ring us up at **icon**, the first question we ask is, "is it hormonally responsive?" Hardly anyone seems to know the answer to this really important question. Go and ask your doctor. If the answer is yes, then there is so much you can do to help yourself. We liken it to an hour glass.

The Top 'Bowl': Consists of changing your eating habits. Smaller meals, 5–6 times a day, less salt, no refined carbohydrate, no insulin rushes, no sugar, fizzy soft drinks. Clean, oestrogen free water. Phytoestrogens, pulses, fruits. Roughage, isoflavones and garlic (which both limit cancer spread). And supplements.

The Centre: Go and talk to an integrated doctor about natural progesterone treatment.

The Lower 'Bowl': Clean up your house; repaint if the paint is over 15 years old; beware chipboard, carpet and ceiling tiles – the glues might be toxic.

Don't put perfumes or perfumed products on your skin, or use talc, or toiletries, cosmetics, creams and toners with toxins in them. (Don't put toxic ingredients near your children.)

Don't breathe toxic gases from bleaches, disinfectants, polishes and cleaners, or petrol fumes. Keep computers and faxes downstairs.

Switch to a supplier of toxin-free products like Neways.

APPENDICES

15 potentially harmful ingredients to avoid – at all costs

(Reproduced from icon magazine)

Is your bathroom cabinet bulging with toxins? Is your make-up or toilet bag a cocktail of chemicals that could do you harm? Yes is probably the answer to both of those questions. The higher up the list of ingredients these 15 come, the greater the concentration. So check your products today, then chuck out and buy safer alternatives.

1   **Formaldehyde** – Combined with water, this toxic gas is used as a disinfectant, fixative, germicide and preservative in deodorants, liquid soaps, nail varnish and shampoos. Also known as formalin, formal and methyl aldehyde, it is a suspected human carcinogen and has caused lung cancer in rats. It can damage DNA, irritate the eyes, upper respiratory tract and mucous membrane, and may cause asthma and headaches. It is banned in Japan and Sweden. Can appear under 50 or so different names in ingredients lists.

2   **Phthalates** – hit the headlines last year for being 'gender benders'. They are a family of industrial 'plasticisers' already banned in the EU from being used in plastic toys, but are still in hairsprays, top-selling perfumes and nail varnishes. You can also ingest them as they leach from PET and soft plastic bottles into your healthy designer water and the kids' fizzy drinks. They can be absorbed through

the skin, inhaled as fumes and ingested from contaminated food or breastfeeding. Animal studies have shown they can damage the liver, kidneys, lungs and reproductive system – especially developing testes.

3   **Parabens** – are listed as alkyl parahydroxy benzoates – butyl/methyl/ethyl/ propyl/isobutyl paraben on some toothpastes, moisturisers, deodorants, antiperspirants and even sunscreens. They are used as a preservative, although some people feel they act as oestrogen mimics. Recent research suggests that parabens in antiperspirant deodorants might cause breast cancer. However, other research suggests parabens are not absorbed through the intestine, and through the skin it is rapidly degraded, while any reaching the blood is quickly hydrolysed. Research has also brought into question any effect on cell receptor sites but none the less parabens accumulate in breast cells and other cancer tissues. So while the jury is out it is best to avoid products containing parabens for now.

4   **Sodium Lauryl Sulphate (SLS)** – is one of the major ingredients in nearly every shampoo, bubble bath, liquid soap etc. Why, when it is a known skin irritant, stops hair growth, can cause cataracts in adults, damage children's eye development and cause urinary tract infection? It's cheap and produces lots of bubbles when mixed with salt. Hardly compensation! Sodium Laureth Sulphate (SLES) is a slightly less irritating form of SLS, but may cause more drying. Both can lead to

potentially carcinogenic cocktails of nitrites and dioxins forming in shampoos and cleansers, by reacting with other ingredients. Most importantly SLS weakens the impermeability of the skin allowing more toxins across and into the blood stream.

5   **Toluene** – is a common solvent found in nail enamels, hair gels, hair spray, and perfumes. It is a neurotoxin and can damage the liver, disrupt the endocrine system and cause asthma.

6   **Alpha Hydroxy Acid** – Long-term skin damage can result from using products containing AHAs (sometimes listed as triple fruit acids, lactic acid, sugar cane extract or glycolic acid). They exfoliate, not only damaged layers of skin but the skin's protective barrier as well. This can decrease protection from the sun by 30 per cent and increase the absorption of chemical ingredients never meant to get through.

7   **Alcohol** – We're talking about the kind found in ingestible products here, like mouthwash. Children have died from accidentally swallowing too much of it. Mouthwashes with an alcohol content of 25 per cent or more have been linked to mouth, tongue and throat cancers.

8   **Propylene Glycol** – is a cosmetic form of mineral oil (refined crude oil) used in industrial antifreeze. People handling it are warned by the manufacturer to avoid skin contact and wear respirators and rubber gloves etc, and yet this is a

major ingredient in most moisturisers, skin creams, baby wipes and sunscreens. Why? It's cheap and gives the 'glide' factor in body lotions – but is in fact robbing lower layers of skin of moisture. Lanolin and collagen also clog pores and cause skin to age faster than if nothing was used.

9   **Talc** – is recognised as carcinogenic, having a similar chemical structure to asbestos, and has been linked to an increased risk of ovarian cancer and general urinary tract disorders. So don't dust it on your baby's, or anyone else's, bottom!

10 **Xylene** – is listed as xytol or dimethylbenzene on nail varnish bottles. It can damage your liver, is narcotic in high concentrations and causes skin and respiratory tract irritation.

11 **Parfum/perfume** – A typical cosmetic can contain up to 100 chemicals in the perfume alone! 95 per cent of these chemicals are synthetic compounds derived from petroleum – 26 of which are on an EU hit list. Fragrances have been linked to allergies and breathing difficulties and they penetrate the skin. The Swedes have research linking perfumed products to high levels of DEHB in body. This is a highy toxic oestrogen mimic.

12 **Diethanolamine** – Also Tri and Mono (DEA, TEA and MEA) are absorbed through skin where they accumulate in organs. When found in products also containing nitrates, they react and form nitrosamines which are carcinogenic.

13 **Aluminium** – is found in most deodorants, has been linked to Alzheimer's, and is increasingly being linked to cancer.

14 **Triclosan** – sometimes listed as 5-chloro-2 (2,4-dichlorophenoxy)-phenol, is in deodorants, toothpastes, vaginal washes and mouthwashes. Toxic dioxins are produced during its manufacture or incineration. It is stored in breast milk and in fish, and can break down in water to create a member of the toxic dioxin family.

15 **Paraphenylenediamine** – or PPD is used in dark hair dyes. Tests on rats have shown that PPD may cause cancer, after long-term use with hydrogen peroxide. It has been implicated in numerous bladder cancer cases in California. The perfect excuse to go blonde?

Call **icon** *on 01280 815166 for more information on safe products.*

As safe as houses?

(Reproduced from icon magazine)

You watch what you eat, you've taken up yoga and you've joined the gym. A few years ago you gave up smoking and moderated your alcohol consumption. So what's the problem? You're doing everything you can to beat the big C. Or are you?

We are all aware of the ever increasing toxins in our environment and trying to beat cancer sometimes resembles running up a down escalator as we try to do our best, for ourselves and our families, against a tidal wave of daily carcinogenic toxins that seem determined to cause us harm. At least we can retreat into the safety of our own homes.

Well, actually, that's where most of the problems start!

Household toxins can seriously damage your children

A toxic environment may be dangerous for us adults, but it is far, far worse for our children. There is abundant evidence that infants and children are far more susceptible to the negative influence of toxins. Experiments with carcinogens on mice (mice share 99 per cent of the same genes as humans) show that some carcinogens have little or no effect on the adult mice, but cause illness and death amongst all the young. Even with active carcinogens by adulthood we seem to build up immunity to many.

Indeed there is also evidence that some problems

actually can start much earlier. Research on oestrogen mimics in perfumes used by pregnant women showed links to a 4 per cent level of testicular cancer in male offspring, according to one Swedish study.

An outside chance

The dangers can start as soon as you walk through the front gate. Moss killers, weed killers, ant killers, rose sprays: if they are harmful to the genes of plants and aphids why would they not be harmful to your genes? The link between cancer and pesticide exposure is well documented. Children under 14 whose gardens have been sprayed with herbicides have a four times greater incidence of connective tissue tumours; pesticides used to eradicate garden insects are linked with increased levels of brain tumours in children in one study and with a four-fold increase in childhood leukaemia in another.

Then you stroke the cat and pat the dog; flea collars may keep the pests away from your house, but they too have been directly linked with increased levels of cancer, especially in children. Pet sprays and shampoos all contain pesticides. Instead try feeding your cat garlic and brewers yeast. Try rubbing the fur with clove or eucalyptus oil. To reduce the garden bugs, look for more organic approaches. Vinegar pots kill slugs, good old fashioned fly paper still works, marigolds keep the aphids off garden vegetables, chickens eat the moth bugs that descend from the apple trees in winter, garlic and onions have a control effect on aphids too, not just vampires!

Spend time in the garden sunshine and without adequate sunscreen you may burn a little. Although your skin cancer might not develop until you reach your sixties, there is ample evidence that it was originally caused in your teens. Slap some sunscreen on and the risk of cancer diminishes.

Er, well not exactly. In 2000 fourteen sunscreen products were banned in Scandinavia because ingredients such as P.A.B.A. and parabens were adjudged to be carcinogenic. Look for the P.A.B.A.-free alternatives. There is even recent research saying that most sunscreens only take out about 80 per cent of UVB rays. And finally many ingredients in our everyday lives can result in oestrogen mimics in our bodies. And higher levels of oestrogen are known to increase skin cancer risk; so the sunshine itself may only be one factor in what is becoming the second largest cancer in the Western world.

Home sweet home

We finally make it to the front door. Here it is a good idea to adopt an oriental custom and leave your outdoor shoes outside. Why walk the germs, pesticides and herbicides into the house and onto the carpets? Again scientific studies have shown that is exactly what you do!

Relax in the lounge and take a deep breath at the end of a tiring day. If the formaldehyde doesn't get you the radon might!

Formaldehyde is a class A (the worst sort) carcinogen present from the manufacture of cheaper woods (plywood and chipboards), and from some fixatives for carpets and tiles. It certainly causes respiratory and eye problems and the FDA in America has stated that it may even cause cancer. Formaldehyde is used to stiffen many fabrics, from new clothing to upholstery and carpets. It is also contained in many cosmetic and skin and personal care products. It is found in household cleaning products, mould and mildew cleaners and even in articles from furniture to contraceptives (see VOCs later in this article). Formaldehyde has over 50 different synonyms used by manufacturers to hide its presence.

So read labels and avoid products containing it; wash all new clothing before wearing it and leave newly carpeted and curtained rooms a week or two with the windows open before you or your children sleep there. Always use 100 per cent cotton sheets and wash them before use.

Radon is an inert gas. You cannot see it, smell it or taste it. It bubbles up through the flooring if your house is on certain types of soil containing even low quantities of uranium. The decomposing uranium gives off radon, which rises into the house. You could try opening all the doors and windows, but this is not wonderfully effective as the radon 'sticks' to dust particles in the localised environment of the house. When you breathe in, these dust particles go to the deepest recesses of your lungs and the radon decomposes further resulting in carcinogenic activity. Don't be under any illusions about this. Several big studies in the USA, and the Surgeon General, have concluded that radon is the second largest cause of lung cancer after cigarette smoking. Indeed, if it combines with cigarette smoking, risks are disproportionately multiplied. The answer is simple, contact the Radiological Protection Board on 0800 614529 or visit www.nrpb.org ideally before you buy the house as pockets of uranium soil, although predominantly in areas of South West England and Wales, exist all over the UK.

Throwing open the windows may not always be the safest thing to do, though. If you live near a main road you are inviting all those nasty **diesel fumes** to enter your home. These work much the same way as radon. They particulate, you breathe them in, and then the toxins in them get to work and attack your lungs. Make no mistake diesel fumes are dangerous and after smoking and radon, diesel fumes are the next biggest cause of lung cancer. Lorries, buses and taxis using diesel, especially those with old and poor exhaust systems are a real danger. (It's a shame manufacturers cannot fit electrostatic exhaust filters as standard to remove particulates and cut emissions.)

Of course, you have given up **smoking**. But have all those around you? Certainly there is compelling evidence to ask visitors and guests not to smoke in your home. Recent research from Cancer Research UK has concluded that the harm from passive smoking is much worse than originally thought. Passive smokers where another person in the same household smokes, breathe six times more smoke per day than non-passive smokers. Females are particularly vulnerable as the risks of smoking link to factors in the airways. These factors are produced by the X chromosome. (In our

DNA each of us has two chromosomes. Women have two X chromosomes and men have an X and a Y. Thus women produce twice as many X related airway factors). Women whose husbands smoke, have almost the same risk of lung cancer as their smoker husbands even though they might not smoke themselves.

Lead is another toxin that can enter through those open windows, although less and less as lead-free petrols are widely used now. However, the soil alongside major roads has been found to still be contaminated, another reason to kick off those shoes at the front door! It has not been proven to be carcinogenic but it is extremely toxic to the nervous system, kidneys, blood system and in cell reproduction. Lead is still found in paints made before 1980. Maybe it's time to brighten up your house. But nowadays lead comes into your home another way – your water system. Many towns still have old lead piping, for example, I know of one house that had blue water from copper pipes!

You are what you drink

Many people will shop organically, cut dairy, eat more vegetables and chant the mantra, 'you are what you eat', before settling down to a nice cup of tea in front of the TV. There is a weird irony about water in the home. Young lycra clad women on running machines have their plastic bottled mineral water about them at all times. A symbol of health, indeed fashion.

Then they cook in tap water, or eat out in restaurants that do the same.

Tap water was covered extensively in **icon** January 2003. It contains chlorine which reacts with organic materials to form highly carcinogenic trihalomethanes, and often fluoride. It contains heavy metals like aluminium and lead and recycled water in major cities contains oestrogen levels you most definitely do not need. Increasingly some tap waters contain chlorine resistant microscopic parasites.

Boiling the water may kill off parasites, bacteria and viruses, but it only serves to concentrate the other impurities, making your organic vegetables very toxic, and your caffeine-free coffee more hazardous than healthy. I saw a test where an electric current was passed between two electrodes in tap water. The charge will only pass if there are impurities. After thirty seconds the water was warm and had turned varying colours of yellow, brown, green and blue. It was not a pretty sight!

The solution is to purchase or rent a reverse osmosis water filter, which will take out all the nasties. Contact **icon** on 01280 815166 for our cost price offer. You consume eight pints of water per day and cook with it as well. You can clean it up completely for less than £5 per week. This has to make sense.

Oestrogen mimics pose a real danger. They add to the body's oestrogen pool, already much higher in 2003 than in 1003. Don't breathe the fumes when you put petrol in the car; don't use plastic bottled water, which leaches phthalates (more oestrogen mimics) from the plastic into the supposedly pure water, remove oestrogen from tap water with a filter, beware perfumes, deodorants, hairsprays and shampoos (see **icon** January 2004 and fuller report in February 2004). The list is seemingly endless.

The ultimate solution

Oestrogen mimics are part of a larger collection of known toxins called volatile organic compounds (VOCs). VOCs comprise hundreds, even thousands of man-made and even natural carbon-based agents.

Toluene, xylene, trichloroethylene and l-trichloro-ethane comprise the majority of the solvent market. VOCs are ideal solvents and are also found in pesticides and disinfectants. If you walk down the cleaner aisle of your grocery store you can smell them in the air. The gases can pass through plastic containers; you absorb them by breathing, ingestion or through absorption via the skin. VOCs have been placed third by the American EPA after cigarette smoke and radon as indoor carcinogens. **EPA statistics show that women working at home have a 55 per cent increased risk of cancer over those who work away from home!**

VOCs are found in paints, varnishes, glues, dyes, cleaning products, inks, perfumes, polish removers and more. The only way to stay safe is to buy these products where possible from companies who make toxin-free alternatives. (Neways is a good example.)

One American scientific study showed that indoor air was actually more polluted than the outdoor air in New York and Los Angeles!

We have talked about formaldehyde, but other harmful substances include:

Phenols: found in disinfectants, air fresheners, furniture polishes and paint removers. But also in fragrances, nail polish, lip balm, antiseptics, lipstick, mouthwashes and other personal care products.

Creosol: found in numerous products from paint removers and disinfectants to personal care products.

Benzene and nitrobenzene; these cross cell walls, damage immune systems and are known carcinogens. Again found in a variety of products from furniture polish to personal care products.

Ammonia: found in cleaners, furniture polish and fabric softeners. But also in antiperspirants, disinfectants, beauty products, personal care and even baby products!

Chlorine: in everything from tap water to bleach and swimming pools and jacuzzis. Chlorine gas was after all a warfare agent. You can remove much of it by cleaning up your drinking water as we said above and using an ozone-producing unit for the jacuzzi.

If you are painting or decorating, keep the area very well ventilated for weeks after the job is finished. Have lots of live plants around especially foliage varieties like spider plants. Cover chipboards and plywoods fast if you can't remove them. Look for manufacturers of 'safer' carpet tiles like Interface.

Become ingredients-conscious; but this is difficult as there are so many names and so much is hidden, so buy toxin-free products wherever possible. Keep the dust down: the more dust in the air the more toxins you inhale as evaporating VOCs and toxins like lead 'stick' to the particles, just like radon and diesel fumes. Perhaps the most worrying thing about these in-home toxins is that it is much easier to believe that nasty smelling household cleaners are more harmful than your carpet. Then you find both are hazards.

Carpets hold over a hundred times more dust than wood flooring and lead levels in carpet dust exceed those in toxic clean-up factory sites! Think about getting rid of your carpets! If not, vacuum at least twice per week and use a vacuum cleaner with a HEPA filter. The interesting thing is 'safer' household products are usually no more expensive than their toxic rivals.

And so to bed

Worse is to come in your bedroom and bathroom.

Have you washed your hands yet? Depending on what you did today your hands could be covered in bad bacteria, or in nickel from coins, or in pesticides and herbicides if you just had a round of golf.

So you wash your hands and brush your teeth. But most soaps and toothpaste contain sodium lauryl sulphate, (also found in shampoos and shower gels). It is used as a wetting agent and apart from providing toxic residues to the heart, lungs, liver and brain (*Journal of American Toxicology* Vol. 2 No. 7 1983), it increases the permeability of the skin by 40 per cent allowing the toxins more freedom of absorption. There is no evidence that sodium lauryl sulphate is carcinogenic but it can cause 'severe' epidermal changes.

So you take a bath, increasing your skin's permeability and bathing yourself in the chlorine, lead, copper and aluminium solution we call water. If you want to make matters worse you could always add bath salts to the bath, especially the perfumed sort! And afterwards men and women alike may dry themselves off and spread a little talc around. Who hasn't used a little on themselves or even the baby's bottom?

According to the US News and World Report (1997, March) talc used in the genital area increases ovarian cancer risk significantly (by 60 per cent or more) whilst **feminine deodorants** increase risk by 90 per cent!

In the USA toothpaste labels actually warn users to contact a poison control center immediately if you swallow any. Have you told your children or grandchildren this? Did you even know?

Now comes the really dangerous part. It's late, cold and the heating kicks in. Downstairs the gas boiler in the kitchen burns away. You may even have cooked with gas. Whilst old appliances, and especially those with a pilot light, are a significant problem, all gas appliances can cause an increase in **nitrogen dioxide** levels in the home. It hasn't been proven as a carcinogen to humans, just to animals, although it is known to significantly impair the immune system and have links to arthritis.

You must vent your kitchen to the outside fully and ideally have the boiler in a room completely outside the house. The by-products of combustion like nitrogen dioxide will rise through your home, ending up in your bedroom and they can exceed maximum limits set for the gas in polluted city centres!

You may not feel tired yet so you stop to tidy up the kid's toys. Many plastic toys contain polyvinyl chloride. In landfill sites this requires special treatment as a toxic waste. Polypropylene and wood are safer alternatives. PVC furniture and coverings (for example, in new car seats) give off carcinogenic gases.

Still not tired, you pop into your office and flick on the computer; you have a fax to read too. VOCs (including benzene) evaporate from the computer circuitry, laser printers and fax machines in operation. Keep all these machines well away from bedrooms and in rooms that are well ventilated at all times. Don't let your children play computer games upstairs.

And so to bed. Blast! The mobile phone goes. You put it to your ear and the ionising radiation floods into your skull. Maybe you use an earpiece; it doesn't matter, the great majority make little difference. Swedish and Finnish research concludes you damage your blood–brain barrier and a few of those toxins in your body are given a chance to get in and poison your brain. (See **icon** November 2002, or www.canceractive.com – 'The case against mobile phones'.) It's for your eight-year-old son who is still awake. He takes the call. His skull is thinner than yours, more vulnerable to the radiation. Research by the *Ecologist*, and Spanish scientists bears this out.

The call is thankfully short, you switch on the TV but there's nothing good on, so off it goes and you get into bed, turning the lights off either side of the bed.

Ah, a nice, warm, bed; at least the electric blanket works.

Have you considered that the cosy glow you feel may be in part due to the surrounding magnetic radiation? From the TV (turned off or on standby), the electrical fields generated by the bedside electricity and the electric blanket.

At least the sheets and pillowcases are cotton, now washed in carcinogen-free products, and the pillows filled with carcinogen-free filling.

If you want to reduce these known carcinogens in your life take the TV and electric blanket from your bedroom and get an electrician to move the bedside wiring. If you have a TV in your bedroom, cover it at night time and unplug it from the mains. This should abolish the electromagnetic field. A team of researchers at the University of San Antonio, Texas linked EMFs to the suppression of melatonin production and thus to an increased cancer risk. Melatonin production peaks about one to two hours after falling asleep, pushing you into a deeper sleep. Melatonin can reduce oestrogen levels and also acts as an excellent neutraliser of free radicals in the body.

Vow to move away from the nearby power lines. Nine studies in the UK show that relatively low levels of EMFs from power cables, pylons or mains electricity are linked to an increase of childhood cancers especially leukaemia. This has been confirmed in Sweden and the USA. Vow to write to the local council about the mobile phone mast they are erecting next door. The Spanish village that won a court case in

2002 successfully drew attention to the childhood cancers in the village since the masts arrived.

Some homes sit on EMF fault lines, or at points of high magnetic fields caused by several transmitters often miles away, yet coinciding.

The UK Radiological Protection Board may be able to help on this one and check out your home.

Ah. To sleep, perchance to dream.

It could have been worse; at least you gave the sun bed a miss and didn't use your old microwave oven!

To order more copies of this book

Tel: 44(0)1280 815166

Fax: 44(0)1280 824655

E-mail: enquiries@iconmag.co.uk

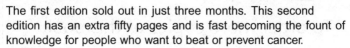

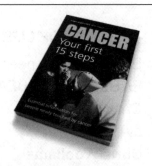

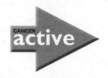